THIS BOOK BELONGS TO :

_____

_____

PATIENT NAME :		**BIRTHDAY:**		**SOC :**		**HT :**
DOCTOR NAME :		**PHONE NUMBER:**				

PMH PRIMARY DIAGNOSIS :

MONTH					
KPS					
PPS					
WEIGHT					
BMI					
AMBUL-ATION					
BATHING					
TRANSFER					
RESPIRATORY					
CARDIAC					
SKIN					

FEEDING (INTAKE)						
SLEEP						
CONTINENCE						
COGNITION						
FALLS						
FAST SCORE						
INFECTIONS						
LABS APPOINTMENTS						

DAY:....../....../.....   HOME HEALTH AID (HHA):

FUNERAL HOME:

PHONE NUMBER:

POA/FAMILY MEMBER AND CONTACT INFO:

NAME:

PHONE NUMBER:

CHECK ALL THAT APPLY :(SEE SUMMARY FOR FURTHER DETAILS)

☐ GLASSES   ☐ COAGS   ☐ DENTURES

☐ HEARING DISABILITY   ☐ DIABETES   ☐ THYROID

PATIENT NAME :		BIRTHDAY:		SOC :	HT :

PATIENT NAME :   BIRTHDAY: SOC :   HT :

DOCTOR NAME :   PHONE NUMBER:

PMH PRIMARY DIAGNOSIS :

MONTH						
KPS						
PPS						
WEIGHT						
BMI						
AMBUL-ATION						
BATHING						
TRANSFER						
RESPIRATORY						
CARDIAC						
SKIN						

FEEDING (INTAKE)						
SLEEP						
CONTINENCE						
COGNITION						
FALLS						
FAST SCORE						
INFECTIONS						
LABS APPOINTMENTS						

DAY:...../...../.....　　　　　　　　HOME HEALTH AID (HHA):

FUNERAL HOME:

POA/FAMILY MEMBER AND CONTACT INFO:　　NAME:

PHONE NUMBER:　　　　　　　　　　PHONE NUMBER:

CHECK ALL THAT APPLY :(SEE SUMMARY FOR FURTHER DETAILS)

☐ GLASSES　　　　　☐ COAGS　　　　　☐ DENTURES

☐ HEARING DISABILITY　　☐ DIABETES　　　☐ THYROID

PATIENT NAME :		**BIRTHDAY:**		**SOC :**		**HT :**
DOCTOR NAME :		**PHONE NUMBER:**				

PMH PRIMARY DIAGNOSIS :

MONTH						
KPS						
PPS						
WEIGHT						
BMI						
AMBUL-ATION						
BATHING						
TRANSFER						
RESPIRATORY						
CARDIAC						
SKIN						

FEEDING (INTAKE)						
SLEEP						
CONTINENCE						
COGNITION						
FALLS						
FAST SCORE						
INFECTIONS						
LABS APPOINTMENTS						

DAY:...../...../.....   HOME HEALTH AID (HHA):

FUNERAL HOME:

PHONE NUMBER:

POA/FAMILY MEMBER AND CONTACT INFO:

NAME:

PHONE NUMBER:

CHECK ALL THAT APPLY :(SEE SUMMARY FOR FURTHER DETAILS)

☐ GLASSES   ☐ COAGS   ☐ DENTURES

☐ HEARING DISABILITY   ☐ DIABETES   ☐ THYROID

PATIENT NAME :		BIRTHDAY:		SOC :		HT :	
DOCTOR NAME :		PHONE NUMBER:					
PMH PRIMARY DIAGNOSIS :							
MONTH							
KPS							
PPS							
WEIGHT							
BMI							
AMBUL- ATION							
BATHING							
TRANSFER							
RESPIRATORY							
CARDIAC							
SKIN							

FEEDING (INTAKE)						
SLEEP						
CONTINENCE						
COGNITION						
FALLS						
FAST SCORE						
INFECTIONS						
LABS APPOINTMENTS						

DAY:...../...../.....   HOME HEALTH AID (HHA):

FUNERAL HOME:	POA/FAMILY MEMBER AND CONTACT INFO:	NAME:
PHONE NUMBER:		PHONE NUMBER:

CHECK ALL THAT APPLY :(SEE SUMMARY FOR FURTHER DETAILS)

- ☐ GLASSES
- ☐ COAGS
- ☐ DENTURES
- ☐ HEARING DISABILITY
- ☐ DIABETES
- ☐ THYROID

PATIENT NAME :		BIRTHDAY:		SOC :		HT :

DOCTOR NAME : **PHONE NUMBER:**

PMH PRIMARY DIAGNOSIS :

MONTH						
KPS						
PPS						
WEIGHT						
BMI						
AMBUL-ATION						
BATHING						
TRANSFER						
RESPIRATORY						
CARDIAC						
SKIN						

FEEDING (INTAKE)						
SLEEP						
CONTINENCE						
COGNITION						
FALLS						
FAST SCORE						
INFECTIONS						
LABS APPOINTMENTS						

DAY:...../...../.....   HOME HEALTH AID (HHA):

FUNERAL HOME:

PHONE NUMBER:

POA/FAMILY MEMBER AND CONTACT INFO:

NAME:

PHONE NUMBER:

CHECK ALL THAT APPLY :(SEE SUMMARY FOR FURTHER DETAILS)

☐ GLASSES   ☐ COAGS   ☐ DENTURES

☐ HEARING DISABILITY   ☐ DIABETES   ☐ THYROID

PATIENT NAME :		BIRTHDAY:		SOC :		HT :
DOCTOR NAME :		PHONE NUMBER:				
PMH PRIMARY DIAGNOSIS :						
MONTH						
KPS						
PPS						
WEIGHT						
BMI						
AMBUL-ATION						
BATHING						
TRANSFER						
RESPIRATORY						
CARDIAC						
SKIN						

FEEDING (INTAKE)						
SLEEP						
CONTINENCE						
COGNITION						
FALLS						
FAST SCORE						
INFECTIONS						
LABS APPOINTMENTS						

DAY:...../...../.....   HOME HEALTH AID (HHA):

FUNERAL HOME:	POA/FAMILY MEMBER AND CONTACT INFO: NAME:
PHONE NUMBER:	PHONE NUMBER:

CHECK ALL THAT APPLY :(SEE SUMMARY FOR FURTHER DETAILS)

☐ GLASSES   ☐ COAGS   ☐ DENTURES

☐ HEARING DISABILITY   ☐ DIABETES   ☐ THYROID

| PATIENT NAME : | | BIRTHDAY: | | SOC : | | HT : |
| DOCTOR NAME : | | PHONE NUMBER: | | | | |

PMH PRIMARY DIAGNOSIS :

MONTH						
KPS						
PPS						
WEIGHT						
BMI						
AMBUL-ATION						
BATHING						
TRANSFER						
RESPIRATORY						
CARDIAC						
SKIN						

FEEDING (INTAKE)						
SLEEP						
CONTINENCE						
COGNITION						
FALLS						
FAST SCORE						
INFECTIONS						
LABS APPOINTMENTS						

DAY:....../....../.....   HOME HEALTH AID (HHA):

FUNERAL HOME: PHONE NUMBER:	POA/FAMILY MEMBER AND CONTACT INFO:	NAME: PHONE NUMBER:

CHECK ALL THAT APPLY :(SEE SUMMARY FOR FURTHER DETAILS)

☐ GLASSES   ☐ COAGS   ☐ DENTURES

☐ HEARING DISABILITY   ☐ DIABETES   ☐ THYROID

PATIENT NAME :		BIRTHDAY:		SOC :		HT :
DOCTOR NAME :		PHONE NUMBER:				
PMH PRIMARY DIAGNOSIS :						
MONTH						
KPS						
PPS						
WEIGHT						
BMI						
AMBUL-ATION						
BATHING						
TRANSFER						
RESPIRATORY						
CARDIAC						
SKIN						

FEEDING (INTAKE)						
SLEEP						
CONTINENCE						
COGNITION						
FALLS						
FAST SCORE						
INFECTIONS						
LABS APPOINTMENTS						

DAY:...../...../.....   HOME HEALTH AID (HHA):

FUNERAL HOME:

PHONE NUMBER:

POA/FAMILY MEMBER AND CONTACT INFO:

NAME:

PHONE NUMBER:

CHECK ALL THAT APPLY :(SEE SUMMARY FOR FURTHER DETAILS)

☐ GLASSES   ☐ COAGS   ☐ DENTURES

☐ HEARING DISABILITY   ☐ DIABETES   ☐ THYROID

PATIENT NAME :		BIRTHDAY:		SOC :	HT :
DOCTOR NAME :		PHONE NUMBER:			
PMH PRIMARY DIAGNOSIS :					
MONTH					
KPS					
PPS					
WEIGHT					
BMI					
AMBUL-ATION					
BATHING					
TRANSFER					
RESPIRATORY					
CARDIAC					
SKIN					

FEEDING (INTAKE)						
SLEEP						
CONTINENCE						
COGNITION						
FALLS						
FAST SCORE						
INFECTIONS						
LABS APPOINTMENTS						

DAY:....../....../......   HOME HEALTH AID (HHA):

FUNERAL HOME:	POA/FAMILY MEMBER AND CONTACT INFO:	NAME:
PHONE NUMBER:		PHONE NUMBER:

CHECK ALL THAT APPLY :(SEE SUMMARY FOR FURTHER DETAILS)

☐ GLASSES   ☐ COAGS   ☐ DENTURES

☐ HEARING DISABILITY   ☐ DIABETES   ☐ THYROID

PATIENT NAME :		BIRTHDAY:		SOC :		HT :
DOCTOR NAME :		PHONE NUMBER:				
PMH PRIMARY DIAGNOSIS :						
MONTH						
KPS						
PPS						
WEIGHT						
BMI						
AMBUL-ATION						
BATHING						
TRANSFER						
RESPIRATORY						
CARDIAC						
SKIN						

FEEDING (INTAKE)						
SLEEP						
CONTINENCE						
COGNITION						
FALLS						
FAST SCORE						
INFECTIONS						
LABS APPOINTMENTS						

DAY:....../....../.....   HOME HEALTH AID (HHA):

FUNERAL HOME:	NAME:
	POA/FAMILY MEMBER AND CONTACT INFO:
PHONE NUMBER:	PHONE NUMBER:

CHECK ALL THAT APPLY :(SEE SUMMARY FOR FURTHER DETAILS)

- ☐ GLASSES
- ☐ COAGS
- ☐ DENTURES
- ☐ HEARING DISABILITY
- ☐ DIABETES
- ☐ THYROID

PATIENT NAME :		BIRTHDAY:		SOC :		HT :
DOCTOR NAME :		PHONE NUMBER:				

PMH PRIMARY DIAGNOSIS :

MONTH					
KPS					
PPS					
WEIGHT					
BMI					
AMBUL-ATION					
BATHING					
TRANSFER					
RESPIRATORY					
CARDIAC					
SKIN					

FEEDING (INTAKE)						
SLEEP						
CONTINENCE						
COGNITION						
FALLS						
FAST SCORE						
INFECTIONS						
LABS APPOINTMENTS						

DAY:...../...../.....   HOME HEALTH AID (HHA):

FUNERAL HOME:

PHONE NUMBER:

POA/FAMILY MEMBER
AND CONTACT INFO:

NAME:

PHONE NUMBER:

CHECK ALL THAT APPLY :(SEE SUMMARY FOR FURTHER DETAILS)

☐ GLASSES   ☐ COAGS   ☐ DENTURES

☐ HEARING
   DISABILITY   ☐ DIABETES   ☐ THYROID

PATIENT NAME :		BIRTHDAY:		SOC :		HT :	
DOCTOR NAME :		PHONE NUMBER:					

PMH PRIMARY DIAGNOSIS :

MONTH						
KPS						
PPS						
WEIGHT						
BMI						
AMBUL-ATION						
BATHING						
TRANSFER						
RESPIRATORY						
CARDIAC						
SKIN						

FEEDING (INTAKE)						
SLEEP						
CONTINENCE						
COGNITION						
FALLS						
FAST SCORE						
INFECTIONS						
LABS APPOINTMENTS						

DAY:...../...../.....   HOME HEALTH AID (HHA):

FUNERAL HOME:	POA/FAMILY MEMBER AND CONTACT INFO:	NAME:
PHONE NUMBER:		PHONE NUMBER:

CHECK ALL THAT APPLY :(SEE SUMMARY FOR FURTHER DETAILS)

☐ GLASSES   ☐ COAGS   ☐ DENTURES

☐ HEARING DISABILITY   ☐ DIABETES   ☐ THYROID

PATIENT NAME :		BIRTHDAY:		SOC :		HT :

DOCTOR NAME : **PHONE NUMBER:**

PMH PRIMARY DIAGNOSIS :

MONTH						
KPS						
PPS						
WEIGHT						
BMI						
AMBUL-ATION						
BATHING						
TRANSFER						
RESPIRATORY						
CARDIAC						
SKIN						

FEEDING (INTAKE)						
SLEEP						
CONTINENCE						
COGNITION						
FALLS						
FAST SCORE						
INFECTIONS						
LABS APPOINTMENTS						

DAY:....../....../......   HOME HEALTH AID (HHA):

FUNERAL HOME:

PHONE NUMBER:

POA/FAMILY MEMBER AND CONTACT INFO:

NAME:

PHONE NUMBER:

CHECK ALL THAT APPLY :(SEE SUMMARY FOR FURTHER DETAILS)

☐ GLASSES ☐ COAGS ☐ DENTURES

☐ HEARING DISABILITY ☐ DIABETES ☐ THYROID

PATIENT NAME :		BIRTHDAY:		SOC :		HT :
DOCTOR NAME :		PHONE NUMBER:				
PMH PRIMARY DIAGNOSIS :						

MONTH						
KPS						
PPS						
WEIGHT						
BMI						
AMBUL-ATION						
BATHING						
TRANSFER						
RESPIRATORY						
CARDIAC						
SKIN						

FEEDING (INTAKE)						
SLEEP						
CONTINENCE						
COGNITION						
FALLS						
FAST SCORE						
INFECTIONS						
LABS APPOINTMENTS						

DAY:...../...../.....   HOME HEALTH AID (HHA):

FUNERAL HOME:

PHONE NUMBER:

POA/FAMILY MEMBER AND CONTACT INFO:

NAME:

PHONE NUMBER:

CHECK ALL THAT APPLY :(SEE SUMMARY FOR FURTHER DETAILS)

☐ GLASSES   ☐ COAGS   ☐ DENTURES

☐ HEARING DISABILITY   ☐ DIABETES   ☐ THYROID

PATIENT NAME :		BIRTHDAY:		SOC :		HT :
DOCTOR NAME :		PHONE NUMBER:				

PMH PRIMARY DIAGNOSIS :

MONTH						
KPS						
PPS						
WEIGHT						
BMI						
AMBUL-ATION						
BATHING						
TRANSFER						
RESPIRATORY						
CARDIAC						
SKIN						

FEEDING (INTAKE)						
SLEEP						
CONTINENCE						
COGNITION						
FALLS						
FAST SCORE						
INFECTIONS						
LABS APPOINTMENTS						

DAY:...../...../.....   HOME HEALTH AID (HHA):

FUNERAL HOME:

PHONE NUMBER:

POA/FAMILY MEMBER AND CONTACT INFO:

NAME:

PHONE NUMBER:

CHECK ALL THAT APPLY :(SEE SUMMARY FOR FURTHER DETAILS)

☐ GLASSES   ☐ COAGS   ☐ DENTURES

☐ HEARING DISABILITY   ☐ DIABETES   ☐ THYROID

PATIENT NAME :		BIRTHDAY:		SOC :	HT :
DOCTOR NAME :		PHONE NUMBER:			
PMH PRIMARY DIAGNOSIS :					

MONTH					
KPS					
PPS					
WEIGHT					
BMI					
AMBUL-ATION					
BATHING					
TRANSFER					
RESPIRATORY					
CARDIAC					
SKIN					

FEEDING (INTAKE)						
SLEEP						
CONTINENCE						
COGNITION						
FALLS						
FAST SCORE						
INFECTIONS						
LABS APPOINTMENTS						

DAY:...../...../.....   HOME HEALTH AID (HHA):

| FUNERAL HOME: | POA/FAMILY MEMBER AND CONTACT INFO: | NAME: |
| PHONE NUMBER: | | PHONE NUMBER: |

CHECK ALL THAT APPLY :(SEE SUMMARY FOR FURTHER DETAILS)

☐ GLASSES ☐ COAGS ☐ DENTURES

☐ HEARING DISABILITY ☐ DIABETES ☐ THYROID

PATIENT NAME :		BIRTHDAY:		SOC :		HT :
DOCTOR NAME :		PHONE NUMBER:				

PMH PRIMARY DIAGNOSIS :

MONTH						
KPS						
PPS						
WEIGHT						
BMI						
AMBUL-ATION						
BATHING						
TRANSFER						
RESPIRATORY						
CARDIAC						
SKIN						

FEEDING (INTAKE)					
SLEEP					
CONTINENCE					
COGNITION					
FALLS					
FAST SCORE					
INFECTIONS					
LABS APPOINTMENTS					

DAY:....../....../.....   HOME HEALTH AID (HHA):

FUNERAL HOME:

PHONE NUMBER:

POA/FAMILY MEMBER AND CONTACT INFO:

NAME:

PHONE NUMBER:

CHECK ALL THAT APPLY :(SEE SUMMARY FOR FURTHER DETAILS)

☐ GLASSES   ☐ COAGS   ☐ DENTURES

☐ HEARING DISABILITY   ☐ DIABETES   ☐ THYROID

PATIENT NAME :		BIRTHDAY:		SOC :		HT :

DOCTOR NAME : **PHONE NUMBER:**

PMH PRIMARY DIAGNOSIS :

MONTH						
KPS						
PPS						
WEIGHT						
BMI						
AMBUL-ATION						
BATHING						
TRANSFER						
RESPIRATORY						
CARDIAC						
SKIN						

FEEDING (INTAKE)					
SLEEP					
CONTINENCE					
COGNITION					
FALLS					
FAST SCORE					
INFECTIONS					
LABS APPOINTMENTS					

DAY:...../...../.....   HOME HEALTH AID (HHA):

FUNERAL HOME:

PHONE NUMBER:

POA/FAMILY MEMBER AND CONTACT INFO:

NAME:

PHONE NUMBER:

CHECK ALL THAT APPLY :(SEE SUMMARY FOR FURTHER DETAILS)

☐ GLASSES   ☐ COAGS   ☐ DENTURES

☐ HEARING DISABILITY   ☐ DIABETES   ☐ THYROID

PATIENT NAME :			BIRTHDAY:		SOC :	HT :
DOCTOR NAME :			PHONE NUMBER:			
PMH PRIMARY DIAGNOSIS :						
MONTH						
KPS						
PPS						
WEIGHT						
BMI						
AMBUL-ATION						
BATHING						
TRANSFER						
RESPIRATORY						
CARDIAC						
SKIN						

FEEDING (INTAKE)						
SLEEP						
CONTINENCE						
COGNITION						
FALLS						
FAST SCORE						
INFECTIONS						
LABS APPOINTMENTS						

DAY:...../...../.....   HOME HEALTH AID (HHA):

FUNERAL HOME:

PHONE NUMBER:

POA/FAMILY MEMBER AND CONTACT INFO:

NAME:

PHONE NUMBER:

CHECK ALL THAT APPLY :(SEE SUMMARY FOR FURTHER DETAILS)

☐ GLASSES   ☐ COAGS   ☐ DENTURES

☐ HEARING DISABILITY   ☐ DIABETES   ☐ THYROID

PATIENT NAME :		BIRTHDAY:		SOC :		HT :
DOCTOR NAME :		PHONE NUMBER:				

PMH PRIMARY DIAGNOSIS :

MONTH						
KPS						
PPS						
WEIGHT						
BMI						
AMBUL-ATION						
BATHING						
TRANSFER						
RESPIRATORY						
CARDIAC						
SKIN						

FEEDING (INTAKE)						
SLEEP						
CONTINENCE						
COGNITION						
FALLS						
FAST SCORE						
INFECTIONS						
LABS APPOINTMENTS						

DAY:...../...../..... HOME HEALTH AID (HHA):

FUNERAL HOME:

PHONE NUMBER:

POA/FAMILY MEMBER AND CONTACT INFO:

NAME:

PHONE NUMBER:

CHECK ALL THAT APPLY :(SEE SUMMARY FOR FURTHER DETAILS)

☐ GLASSES   ☐ COAGS   ☐ DENTURES

☐ HEARING DISABILITY   ☐ DIABETES   ☐ THYROID

PATIENT NAME :		BIRTHDAY:		SOC :	HT :
DOCTOR NAME :		PHONE NUMBER:			
PMH PRIMARY DIAGNOSIS :					
MONTH					
KPS					
PPS					
WEIGHT					
BMI					
AMBUL-ATION					
BATHING					
TRANSFER					
RESPIRATORY					
CARDIAC					
SKIN					

FEEDING (INTAKE)						
SLEEP						
CONTINENCE						
COGNITION						
FALLS						
FAST SCORE						
INFECTIONS						
LABS APPOINTMENTS						

DAY:...../...../.....   HOME HEALTH AID (HHA):

FUNERAL HOME:

PHONE NUMBER:

POA/FAMILY MEMBER AND CONTACT INFO:

NAME:

PHONE NUMBER:

CHECK ALL THAT APPLY :(SEE SUMMARY FOR FURTHER DETAILS)

☐ GLASSES   ☐ COAGS   ☐ DENTURES

☐ HEARING DISABILITY   ☐ DIABETES   ☐ THYROID

PATIENT NAME :		BIRTHDAY:		SOC :		HT :
DOCTOR NAME :		PHONE NUMBER:				
PMH PRIMARY DIAGNOSIS :						

MONTH						
KPS						
PPS						
WEIGHT						
BMI						
AMBUL-ATION						
BATHING						
TRANSFER						
RESPIRATORY						
CARDIAC						
SKIN						

FEEDING (INTAKE)					
SLEEP					
CONTINENCE					
COGNITION					
FALLS					
FAST SCORE					
INFECTIONS					
LABS APPOINTMENTS					

DAY:....../....../.....   HOME HEALTH AID (HHA):

FUNERAL HOME:

PHONE NUMBER:

POA/FAMILY MEMBER AND CONTACT INFO:

NAME:

PHONE NUMBER:

CHECK ALL THAT APPLY :(SEE SUMMARY FOR FURTHER DETAILS)

☐ GLASSES   ☐ COAGS   ☐ DENTURES

☐ HEARING DISABILITY   ☐ DIABETES   ☐ THYROID

PATIENT NAME :		BIRTHDAY:		SOC :	HT :
DOCTOR NAME :		PHONE NUMBER:			
PMH PRIMARY DIAGNOSIS :					
MONTH					
KPS					
PPS					
WEIGHT					
BMI					
AMBUL-ATION					
BATHING					
TRANSFER					
RESPIRATORY					
CARDIAC					
SKIN					

FEEDING (INTAKE)					
SLEEP					
CONTINENCE					
COGNITION					
FALLS					
FAST SCORE					
INFECTIONS					
LABS APPOINTMENTS					

DAY:...../...../.....   HOME HEALTH AID (HHA):

FUNERAL HOME:

PHONE NUMBER:

POA/FAMILY MEMBER AND CONTACT INFO:

NAME:

PHONE NUMBER:

CHECK ALL THAT APPLY :(SEE SUMMARY FOR FURTHER DETAILS)

☐ GLASSES   ☐ COAGS   ☐ DENTURES

☐ HEARING DISABILITY   ☐ DIABETES   ☐ THYROID

PATIENT NAME :		BIRTHDAY:		SOC :		HT :
DOCTOR NAME :		PHONE NUMBER:				
PMH PRIMARY DIAGNOSIS :						

MONTH						
KPS						
PPS						
WEIGHT						
BMI						
AMBUL-ATION						
BATHING						
TRANSFER						
RESPIRATORY						
CARDIAC						
SKIN						

FEEDING (INTAKE)						
SLEEP						
CONTINENCE						
COGNITION						
FALLS						
FAST SCORE						
INFECTIONS						
LABS APPOINTMENTS						

DAY:...../...../.....   HOME HEALTH AID (HHA):

FUNERAL HOME: **PHONE NUMBER:**	**POA/FAMILY MEMBER AND CONTACT INFO:** **NAME:** **PHONE NUMBER:**

CHECK ALL THAT APPLY :(SEE SUMMARY FOR FURTHER DETAILS)

☐ GLASSES   ☐ COAGS   ☐ DENTURES

☐ HEARING DISABILITY   ☐ DIABETES   ☐ THYROID

PATIENT NAME :		BIRTHDAY:		SOC :		HT :
DOCTOR NAME :		PHONE NUMBER:				

PMH PRIMARY DIAGNOSIS :

MONTH						
KPS						
PPS						
WEIGHT						
BMI						
AMBUL- ATION						
BATHING						
TRANSFER						
RESPIRATORY						
CARDIAC						
SKIN						

FEEDING (INTAKE)						
SLEEP						
CONTINENCE						
COGNITION						
FALLS						
FAST SCORE						
INFECTIONS						
LABS APPOINTMENTS						

DAY:...../...../.....   HOME HEALTH AID (HHA):

FUNERAL HOME:	**POA/FAMILY MEMBER AND CONTACT INFO:** NAME:
PHONE NUMBER:	PHONE NUMBER:

CHECK ALL THAT APPLY :(SEE SUMMARY FOR FURTHER DETAILS)

☐ GLASSES   ☐ COAGS   ☐ DENTURES

☐ HEARING DISABILITY   ☐ DIABETES   ☐ THYROID

PATIENT NAME :		BIRTHDAY:		SOC :		HT :

DOCTOR NAME :   PHONE NUMBER:

PMH PRIMARY DIAGNOSIS :

MONTH						
KPS						
PPS						
WEIGHT						
BMI						
AMBUL-ATION						
BATHING						
TRANSFER						
RESPIRATORY						
CARDIAC						
SKIN						

FEEDING (INTAKE)					
SLEEP					
CONTINENCE					
COGNITION					
FALLS					
FAST SCORE					
INFECTIONS					
LABS APPOINTMENTS					

DAY:...../...../.....   HOME HEALTH AID (HHA):

FUNERAL HOME:

PHONE NUMBER:

POA/FAMILY MEMBER AND CONTACT INFO:

NAME:

PHONE NUMBER:

CHECK ALL THAT APPLY :(SEE SUMMARY FOR FURTHER DETAILS)

☐ GLASSES   ☐ COAGS   ☐ DENTURES

☐ HEARING DISABILITY   ☐ DIABETES   ☐ THYROID

| PATIENT NAME : | BIRTHDAY: | SOC : | HT : |
| DOCTOR NAME : | PHONE NUMBER: | | |

PMH PRIMARY DIAGNOSIS :

MONTH						
KPS						
PPS						
WEIGHT						
BMI						
AMBUL-ATION						
BATHING						
TRANSFER						
RESPIRATORY						
CARDIAC						
SKIN						

FEEDING (INTAKE)						
SLEEP						
CONTINENCE						
COGNITION						
FALLS						
FAST SCORE						
INFECTIONS						
LABS APPOINTMENTS						

DAY:...../...../.....   HOME HEALTH AID (HHA):

FUNERAL HOME:

PHONE NUMBER:

POA/FAMILY MEMBER AND CONTACT INFO:

NAME:

PHONE NUMBER:

CHECK ALL THAT APPLY :(SEE SUMMARY FOR FURTHER DETAILS)

☐ GLASSES   ☐ COAGS   ☐ DENTURES

☐ HEARING DISABILITY   ☐ DIABETES   ☐ THYROID

PATIENT NAME :		BIRTHDAY:		SOC :		HT :
DOCTOR NAME :		PHONE NUMBER:				

PMH PRIMARY DIAGNOSIS :

MONTH						
KPS						
PPS						
WEIGHT						
BMI						
AMBUL-ATION						
BATHING						
TRANSFER						
RESPIRATORY						
CARDIAC						
SKIN						

FEEDING (INTAKE)					
SLEEP					
CONTINENCE					
COGNITION					
FALLS					
FAST SCORE					
INFECTIONS					
LABS APPOINTMENTS					

DAY:...../...../.....   HOME HEALTH AID (HHA):

FUNERAL HOME:

PHONE NUMBER:

POA/FAMILY MEMBER AND CONTACT INFO:

NAME:

PHONE NUMBER:

CHECK ALL THAT APPLY :(SEE SUMMARY FOR FURTHER DETAILS)

☐ GLASSES   ☐ COAGS   ☐ DENTURES

☐ HEARING DISABILITY   ☐ DIABETES   ☐ THYROID

PATIENT NAME :		BIRTHDAY:		SOC :	HT :
DOCTOR NAME :		PHONE NUMBER:			
PMH PRIMARY DIAGNOSIS :					
MONTH					
KPS					
PPS					
WEIGHT					
BMI					
AMBUL-ATION					
BATHING					
TRANSFER					
RESPIRATORY					
CARDIAC					
SKIN					

FEEDING (INTAKE)					
SLEEP					
CONTINENCE					
COGNITION					
FALLS					
FAST SCORE					
INFECTIONS					
LABS APPOINTMENTS					

DAY:...../...../.....   HOME HEALTH AID (HHA):

FUNERAL HOME:

PHONE NUMBER:

POA/FAMILY MEMBER AND CONTACT INFO:

NAME:

PHONE NUMBER:

CHECK ALL THAT APPLY :(SEE SUMMARY FOR FURTHER DETAILS)

☐ GLASSES   ☐ COAGS   ☐ DENTURES

☐ HEARING DISABILITY   ☐ DIABETES   ☐ THYROID

PATIENT NAME :		BIRTHDAY:		SOC :		HT :
DOCTOR NAME :		PHONE NUMBER:				
PMH PRIMARY DIAGNOSIS :						

MONTH						
KPS						
PPS						
WEIGHT						
BMI						
AMBUL-ATION						
BATHING						
TRANSFER						
RESPIRATORY						
CARDIAC						
SKIN						

FEEDING (INTAKE)						
SLEEP						
CONTINENCE						
COGNITION						
FALLS						
FAST SCORE						
INFECTIONS						
LABS APPOINTMENTS						

DAY:....../....../.....   HOME HEALTH AID (HHA):

FUNERAL HOME:	NAME:
	POA/FAMILY MEMBER AND CONTACT INFO:
PHONE NUMBER:	PHONE NUMBER:

CHECK ALL THAT APPLY :(SEE SUMMARY FOR FURTHER DETAILS)

☐ GLASSES   ☐ COAGS   ☐ DENTURES

☐ HEARING DISABILITY   ☐ DIABETES   ☐ THYROID

| PATIENT NAME : | | BIRTHDAY: | | SOC : | | HT : |

PATIENT NAME :   **BIRTHDAY:**   **SOC :**   **HT :**

DOCTOR NAME :   **PHONE NUMBER:**

PMH PRIMARY DIAGNOSIS :

MONTH					
KPS					
PPS					
WEIGHT					
BMI					
AMBUL-ATION					
BATHING					
TRANSFER					
RESPIRATORY					
CARDIAC					
SKIN					

FEEDING (INTAKE)						
SLEEP						
CONTINENCE						
COGNITION						
FALLS						
FAST SCORE						
INFECTIONS						
LABS APPOINTMENTS						

DAY:...../...../.....   HOME HEALTH AID (HHA):

FUNERAL HOME:

PHONE NUMBER:

POA/FAMILY MEMBER AND CONTACT INFO:

NAME:

PHONE NUMBER:

CHECK ALL THAT APPLY :(SEE SUMMARY FOR FURTHER DETAILS)

☐ GLASSES   ☐ COAGS   ☐ DENTURES

☐ HEARING DISABILITY   ☐ DIABETES   ☐ THYROID

PATIENT NAME :		BIRTHDAY:		SOC :		HT :	
DOCTOR NAME :		PHONE NUMBER:					

PMH PRIMARY DIAGNOSIS :

MONTH						
KPS						
PPS						
WEIGHT						
BMI						
AMBUL-ATION						
BATHING						
TRANSFER						
RESPIRATORY						
CARDIAC						
SKIN						

FEEDING (INTAKE)					
SLEEP					
CONTINENCE					
COGNITION					
FALLS					
FAST SCORE					
INFECTIONS					
LABS APPOINTMENTS					

DAY:...../...../.....   HOME HEALTH AID (HHA):

FUNERAL HOME:	POA/FAMILY MEMBER AND CONTACT INFO:	NAME:
PHONE NUMBER:		PHONE NUMBER:

CHECK ALL THAT APPLY :(SEE SUMMARY FOR FURTHER DETAILS)

- ☐ GLASSES
- ☐ HEARING DISABILITY
- ☐ COAGS
- ☐ DIABETES
- ☐ DENTURES
- ☐ THYROID

PATIENT NAME :		BIRTHDAY:		SOC :		HT :
DOCTOR NAME :		PHONE NUMBER:				

PMH PRIMARY DIAGNOSIS :

MONTH						
KPS						
PPS						
WEIGHT						
BMI						
AMBUL-ATION						
BATHING						
TRANSFER						
RESPIRATORY						
CARDIAC						
SKIN						

FEEDING (INTAKE)						
SLEEP						
CONTINENCE						
COGNITION						
FALLS						
FAST SCORE						
INFECTIONS						
LABS APPOINTMENTS						

DAY:...../...../.....   HOME HEALTH AID (HHA):

FUNERAL HOME:	POA/FAMILY MEMBER AND CONTACT INFO:	NAME:
PHONE NUMBER:		PHONE NUMBER:

CHECK ALL THAT APPLY :(SEE SUMMARY FOR FURTHER DETAILS)

- ☐ GLASSES
- ☐ HEARING DISABILITY
- ☐ COAGS
- ☐ DIABETES
- ☐ DENTURES
- ☐ THYROID

PATIENT NAME :		BIRTHDAY:		SOC :		HT :
DOCTOR NAME :		PHONE NUMBER:				
PMH PRIMARY DIAGNOSIS :						

MONTH						
KPS						
PPS						
WEIGHT						
BMI						
AMBUL-ATION						
BATHING						
TRANSFER						
RESPIRATORY						
CARDIAC						
SKIN						

FEEDING (INTAKE)					
SLEEP					
CONTINENCE					
COGNITION					
FALLS					
FAST SCORE					
INFECTIONS					
LABS APPOINTMENTS					

DAY:...../...../.....   HOME HEALTH AID (HHA):

FUNERAL HOME: PHONE NUMBER:	POA/FAMILY MEMBER AND CONTACT INFO:	NAME: PHONE NUMBER:

CHECK ALL THAT APPLY :(SEE SUMMARY FOR FURTHER DETAILS)

☐ GLASSES   ☐ COAGS   ☐ DENTURES

☐ HEARING DISABILITY   ☐ DIABETES   ☐ THYROID

PATIENT NAME :		BIRTHDAY:		SOC :		HT :
DOCTOR NAME :		PHONE NUMBER:				

PMH PRIMARY DIAGNOSIS :

MONTH						
KPS						
PPS						
WEIGHT						
BMI						
AMBUL-ATION						
BATHING						
TRANSFER						
RESPIRATORY						
CARDIAC						
SKIN						

FEEDING (INTAKE)						
SLEEP						
CONTINENCE						
COGNITION						
FALLS						
FAST SCORE						
INFECTIONS						
LABS APPOINTMENTS						

DAY:...../...../.....   HOME HEALTH AID (HHA):

FUNERAL HOME:

PHONE NUMBER:

POA/FAMILY MEMBER AND CONTACT INFO:

NAME:

PHONE NUMBER:

CHECK ALL THAT APPLY :(SEE SUMMARY FOR FURTHER DETAILS)

☐ GLASSES ☐ COAGS ☐ DENTURES

☐ HEARING DISABILITY ☐ DIABETES ☐ THYROID

PATIENT NAME :		BIRTHDAY:		SOC :	HT :
DOCTOR NAME :		PHONE NUMBER:			
PMH PRIMARY DIAGNOSIS :					

MONTH					
KPS					
PPS					
WEIGHT					
BMI					
AMBUL-ATION					
BATHING					
TRANSFER					
RESPIRATORY					
CARDIAC					
SKIN					

FEEDING (INTAKE)						
SLEEP						
CONTINENCE						
COGNITION						
FALLS						
FAST SCORE						
INFECTIONS						
LABS APPOINTMENTS						

DAY:...../...../.....   HOME HEALTH AID (HHA):

FUNERAL HOME:

PHONE NUMBER:

POA/FAMILY MEMBER AND CONTACT INFO:

NAME:

PHONE NUMBER:

CHECK ALL THAT APPLY :(SEE SUMMARY FOR FURTHER DETAILS)

☐ GLASSES   ☐ COAGS   ☐ DENTURES

☐ HEARING DISABILITY   ☐ DIABETES   ☐ THYROID

PATIENT NAME :		**BIRTHDAY:**		**SOC :**		**HT :**
DOCTOR NAME :		**PHONE NUMBER:**				

PMH PRIMARY DIAGNOSIS :

MONTH					
KPS					
PPS					
WEIGHT					
BMI					
AMBUL-ATION					
BATHING					
TRANSFER					
RESPIRATORY					
CARDIAC					
SKIN					

FEEDING (INTAKE)					
SLEEP					
CONTINENCE					
COGNITION					
FALLS					
FAST SCORE					
INFECTIONS					
LABS APPOINTMENTS					

DAY:...../...../.....   HOME HEALTH AID (HHA):

FUNERAL HOME:

PHONE NUMBER:

POA/FAMILY MEMBER AND CONTACT INFO:

NAME:

PHONE NUMBER:

CHECK ALL THAT APPLY :(SEE SUMMARY FOR FURTHER DETAILS)

☐ GLASSES   ☐ COAGS   ☐ DENTURES

☐ HEARING DISABILITY   ☐ DIABETES   ☐ THYROID

PATIENT NAME :		BIRTHDAY:		SOC :		HT :
DOCTOR NAME :		PHONE NUMBER:				
PMH PRIMARY DIAGNOSIS :						
MONTH						
KPS						
PPS						
WEIGHT						
BMI						
AMBUL-ATION						
BATHING						
TRANSFER						
RESPIRATORY						
CARDIAC						
SKIN						

FEEDING (INTAKE)					
SLEEP					
CONTINENCE					
COGNITION					
FALLS					
FAST SCORE					
INFECTIONS					
LABS APPOINTMENTS					

DAY:...../...../.....   HOME HEALTH AID (HHA):

FUNERAL HOME:

PHONE NUMBER:

POA/FAMILY MEMBER AND CONTACT INFO:

NAME:

PHONE NUMBER:

CHECK ALL THAT APPLY :(SEE SUMMARY FOR FURTHER DETAILS)

☐ GLASSES   ☐ COAGS   ☐ DENTURES

☐ HEARING DISABILITY   ☐ DIABETES   ☐ THYROID

| PATIENT NAME : | | BIRTHDAY: | | SOC : | | HT : |

| DOCTOR NAME : | | PHONE NUMBER: | | | | |

PMH PRIMARY DIAGNOSIS :

MONTH						
KPS						
PPS						
WEIGHT						
BMI						
AMBUL-ATION						
BATHING						
TRANSFER						
RESPIRATORY						
CARDIAC						
SKIN						

FEEDING (INTAKE)						
SLEEP						
CONTINENCE						
COGNITION						
FALLS						
FAST SCORE						
INFECTIONS						
LABS APPOINTMENTS						

DAY:...../...../.....   HOME HEALTH AID (HHA):

FUNERAL HOME:

PHONE NUMBER:

POA/FAMILY MEMBER AND CONTACT INFO:

NAME:

PHONE NUMBER:

CHECK ALL THAT APPLY :(SEE SUMMARY FOR FURTHER DETAILS)

☐ GLASSES   ☐ COAGS   ☐ DENTURES

☐ HEARING DISABILITY   ☐ DIABETES   ☐ THYROID

PATIENT NAME :		BIRTHDAY:		SOC :		HT :
DOCTOR NAME :		PHONE NUMBER:				
PMH PRIMARY DIAGNOSIS :						

MONTH						
KPS						
PPS						
WEIGHT						
BMI						
AMBUL-ATION						
BATHING						
TRANSFER						
RESPIRATORY						
CARDIAC						
SKIN						

FEEDING (INTAKE)					
SLEEP					
CONTINENCE					
COGNITION					
FALLS					
FAST SCORE					
INFECTIONS					
LABS APPOINTMENTS					

DAY:....../....../.....   HOME HEALTH AID (HHA):

FUNERAL HOME:

PHONE NUMBER:

POA/FAMILY MEMBER AND CONTACT INFO:

NAME:

PHONE NUMBER:

CHECK ALL THAT APPLY :(SEE SUMMARY FOR FURTHER DETAILS)

☐ GLASSES   ☐ COAGS   ☐ DENTURES

☐ HEARING DISABILITY   ☐ DIABETES   ☐ THYROID

| PATIENT NAME : | | BIRTHDAY: | | SOC : | | HT : |
| DOCTOR NAME : | | PHONE NUMBER: | | | | |

PMH PRIMARY DIAGNOSIS :

MONTH						
KPS						
PPS						
WEIGHT						
BMI						
AMBUL-ATION						
BATHING						
TRANSFER						
RESPIRATORY						
CARDIAC						
SKIN						

FEEDING (INTAKE)						
SLEEP						
CONTINENCE						
COGNITION						
FALLS						
FAST SCORE						
INFECTIONS						
LABS APPOINTMENTS						

DAY:...../...../.....   HOME HEALTH AID (HHA):

FUNERAL HOME:

PHONE NUMBER:

POA/FAMILY MEMBER AND CONTACT INFO:

NAME:

PHONE NUMBER:

CHECK ALL THAT APPLY :(SEE SUMMARY FOR FURTHER DETAILS)

☐ GLASSES   ☐ COAGS   ☐ DENTURES

☐ HEARING DISABILITY   ☐ DIABETES   ☐ THYROID

PATIENT NAME :			BIRTHDAY:		SOC :	HT :
DOCTOR NAME :			PHONE NUMBER:			
PMH PRIMARY DIAGNOSIS :						
MONTH						
KPS						
PPS						
WEIGHT						
BMI						
AMBUL- ATION						
BATHING						
TRANSFER						
RESPIRATORY						
CARDIAC						
SKIN						

FEEDING (INTAKE)					
SLEEP					
CONTINENCE					
COGNITION					
FALLS					
FAST SCORE					
INFECTIONS					
LABS APPOINTMENTS					

DAY:...../...../.....   HOME HEALTH AID (HHA):

FUNERAL HOME:

PHONE NUMBER:

POA/FAMILY MEMBER AND CONTACT INFO:

NAME:

PHONE NUMBER:

CHECK ALL THAT APPLY :(SEE SUMMARY FOR FURTHER DETAILS)

☐ GLASSES   ☐ COAGS   ☐ DENTURES

☐ HEARING DISABILITY   ☐ DIABETES   ☐ THYROID

PATIENT NAME :		**BIRTHDAY:**		**SOC :**		**HT :**
DOCTOR NAME :		**PHONE NUMBER:**				

PMH PRIMARY DIAGNOSIS :

MONTH					
KPS					
PPS					
WEIGHT					
BMI					
AMBUL-ATION					
BATHING					
TRANSFER					
RESPIRATORY					
CARDIAC					
SKIN					

FEEDING (INTAKE)						
SLEEP						
CONTINENCE						
COGNITION						
FALLS						
FAST SCORE						
INFECTIONS						
LABS APPOINTMENTS						

DAY:...../...../.....   HOME HEALTH AID (HHA):

FUNERAL HOME:

PHONE NUMBER:

POA/FAMILY MEMBER AND CONTACT INFO:

NAME:

PHONE NUMBER:

CHECK ALL THAT APPLY : (SEE SUMMARY FOR FURTHER DETAILS)

- ☐ GLASSES
- ☐ HEARING DISABILITY
- ☐ COAGS
- ☐ DIABETES
- ☐ DENTURES
- ☐ THYROID

PATIENT NAME :		BIRTHDAY:		SOC :		HT :
DOCTOR NAME :		PHONE NUMBER:				

PMH PRIMARY DIAGNOSIS :

MONTH						
KPS						
PPS						
WEIGHT						
BMI						
AMBUL-ATION						
BATHING						
TRANSFER						
RESPIRATORY						
CARDIAC						
SKIN						

FEEDING (INTAKE)					
SLEEP					
CONTINENCE					
COGNITION					
FALLS					
FAST SCORE					
INFECTIONS					
LABS APPOINTMENTS					

DAY:...../...../.....   HOME HEALTH AID (HHA):

FUNERAL HOME:

PHONE NUMBER:

POA/FAMILY MEMBER AND CONTACT INFO:

NAME:

PHONE NUMBER:

CHECK ALL THAT APPLY :(SEE SUMMARY FOR FURTHER DETAILS)

☐ GLASSES   ☐ COAGS   ☐ DENTURES

☐ HEARING DISABILITY   ☐ DIABETES   ☐ THYROID

	PATIENT NAME :		BIRTHDAY:		SOC :	HT :
	DOCTOR NAME :		PHONE NUMBER:			

PMH PRIMARY DIAGNOSIS :						
MONTH						
KPS						
PPS						
WEIGHT						
BMI						
AMBUL-ATION						
BATHING						
TRANSFER						
RESPIRATORY						
CARDIAC						
SKIN						

FEEDING (INTAKE)						
SLEEP						
CONTINENCE						
COGNITION						
FALLS						
FAST SCORE						
INFECTIONS						
LABS APPOINTMENTS						

DAY:...../...../.....   HOME HEALTH AID (HHA):

FUNERAL HOME:

PHONE NUMBER:

POA/FAMILY MEMBER AND CONTACT INFO:

NAME:

PHONE NUMBER:

CHECK ALL THAT APPLY :(SEE SUMMARY FOR FURTHER DETAILS)

☐ GLASSES   ☐ COAGS   ☐ DENTURES

☐ HEARING DISABILITY   ☐ DIABETES   ☐ THYROID

PATIENT NAME :		BIRTHDAY:		SOC :		HT :
DOCTOR NAME :		PHONE NUMBER:				

PMH PRIMARY DIAGNOSIS :

MONTH						
KPS						
PPS						
WEIGHT						
BMI						
AMBUL-ATION						
BATHING						
TRANSFER						
RESPIRATORY						
CARDIAC						
SKIN						

FEEDING (INTAKE)						
SLEEP						
CONTINENCE						
COGNITION						
FALLS						
FAST SCORE						
INFECTIONS						
LABS APPOINTMENTS						

DAY:...../...../.....   HOME HEALTH AID (HHA):

FUNERAL HOME:	POA/FAMILY MEMBER AND CONTACT INFO:	NAME:
PHONE NUMBER:		PHONE NUMBER:

CHECK ALL THAT APPLY :(SEE SUMMARY FOR FURTHER DETAILS)

☐ GLASSES ☐ COAGS ☐ DENTURES

☐ HEARING DISABILITY ☐ DIABETES ☐ THYROID

| PATIENT NAME : | | BIRTHDAY: | | SOC : | | HT : |
| DOCTOR NAME : | | PHONE NUMBER: | | | | |

PMH PRIMARY DIAGNOSIS :

MONTH						
KPS						
PPS						
WEIGHT						
BMI						
AMBUL-ATION						
BATHING						
TRANSFER						
RESPIRATORY						
CARDIAC						
SKIN						

FEEDING (INTAKE)						
SLEEP						
CONTINENCE						
COGNITION						
FALLS						
FAST SCORE						
INFECTIONS						
LABS APPOINTMENTS						

DAY:...../...../.....   HOME HEALTH AID (HHA):

FUNERAL HOME:	POA/FAMILY MEMBER AND CONTACT INFO:	NAME:
PHONE NUMBER:		PHONE NUMBER:

CHECK ALL THAT APPLY :(SEE SUMMARY FOR FURTHER DETAILS)

- ☐ GLASSES
- ☐ HEARING DISABILITY
- ☐ COAGS
- ☐ DIABETES
- ☐ DENTURES
- ☐ THYROID

| PATIENT NAME : | | BIRTHDAY: | | SOC : | | HT : |
| DOCTOR NAME : | | PHONE NUMBER: | | | | |

PMH PRIMARY DIAGNOSIS :

MONTH						
KPS						
PPS						
WEIGHT						
BMI						
AMBUL-ATION						
BATHING						
TRANSFER						
RESPIRATORY						
CARDIAC						
SKIN						

FEEDING (INTAKE)					
SLEEP					
CONTINENCE					
COGNITION					
FALLS					
FAST SCORE					
INFECTIONS					
LABS APPOINTMENTS					

DAY:...../...../.....   HOME HEALTH AID (HHA):

FUNERAL HOME: PHONE NUMBER:	POA/FAMILY MEMBER AND CONTACT INFO:	NAME: PHONE NUMBER:

CHECK ALL THAT APPLY :(SEE SUMMARY FOR FURTHER DETAILS)

☐ GLASSES   ☐ COAGS   ☐ DENTURES

☐ HEARING DISABILITY   ☐ DIABETES   ☐ THYROID

PATIENT NAME :		BIRTHDAY:		SOC :	HT :
DOCTOR NAME :		PHONE NUMBER:			
PMH PRIMARY DIAGNOSIS :					
MONTH					
KPS					
PPS					
WEIGHT					
BMI					
AMBUL-ATION					
BATHING					
TRANSFER					
RESPIRATORY					
CARDIAC					
SKIN					

FEEDING (INTAKE)						
SLEEP						
CONTINENCE						
COGNITION						
FALLS						
FAST SCORE						
INFECTIONS						
LABS APPOINTMENTS						

DAY:...../...../.....   HOME HEALTH AID (HHA):

FUNERAL HOME:

PHONE NUMBER:

POA/FAMILY MEMBER AND CONTACT INFO:

NAME:

PHONE NUMBER:

CHECK ALL THAT APPLY :(SEE SUMMARY FOR FURTHER DETAILS)

☐ GLASSES   ☐ COAGS   ☐ DENTURES

☐ HEARING DISABILITY   ☐ DIABETES   ☐ THYROID

PATIENT NAME :   BIRTHDAY: SOC :   HT :

DOCTOR NAME :   PHONE NUMBER:

PMH PRIMARY DIAGNOSIS :

MONTH						
KPS						
PPS						
WEIGHT						
BMI						
AMBUL-ATION						
BATHING						
TRANSFER						
RESPIRATORY						
CARDIAC						
SKIN						

FEEDING (INTAKE)					
SLEEP					
CONTINENCE					
COGNITION					
FALLS					
FAST SCORE					
INFECTIONS					
LABS APPOINTMENTS					

DAY:...../...../.....   HOME HEALTH AID (HHA):

FUNERAL HOME:	NAME:
	POA/FAMILY MEMBER AND CONTACT INFO:
PHONE NUMBER:	PHONE NUMBER:

CHECK ALL THAT APPLY :(SEE SUMMARY FOR FURTHER DETAILS)

☐ GLASSES   ☐ COAGS   ☐ DENTURES

☐ HEARING DISABILITY   ☐ DIABETES   ☐ THYROID

| PATIENT NAME : | | BIRTHDAY: | | SOC : | | HT : |
| DOCTOR NAME : | | PHONE NUMBER: | | | | |

PMH PRIMARY DIAGNOSIS :

MONTH						
KPS						
PPS						
WEIGHT						
BMI						
AMBUL-ATION						
BATHING						
TRANSFER						
RESPIRATORY						
CARDIAC						
SKIN						

FEEDING (INTAKE)						
SLEEP						
CONTINENCE						
COGNITION						
FALLS						
FAST SCORE						
INFECTIONS						
LABS APPOINTMENTS						

DAY:...../...../.....   HOME HEALTH AID (HHA):

FUNERAL HOME: PHONE NUMBER:	POA/FAMILY MEMBER AND CONTACT INFO: NAME: PHONE NUMBER:

CHECK ALL THAT APPLY :(SEE SUMMARY FOR FURTHER DETAILS)

☐ GLASSES   ☐ COAGS   ☐ DENTURES

☐ HEARING DISABILITY   ☐ DIABETES   ☐ THYROID

| PATIENT NAME : | | BIRTHDAY: | | SOC : | | HT : |

PATIENT NAME :   BIRTHDAY: SOC :   HT :

DOCTOR NAME :   PHONE NUMBER:

PMH PRIMARY DIAGNOSIS :

MONTH						
KPS						
PPS						
WEIGHT						
BMI						
AMBUL-ATION						
BATHING						
TRANSFER						
RESPIRATORY						
CARDIAC						
SKIN						

FEEDING (INTAKE)					
SLEEP					
CONTINENCE					
COGNITION					
FALLS					
FAST SCORE					
INFECTIONS					
LABS APPOINTMENTS					

DAY:...../...../.....   HOME HEALTH AID (HHA):

FUNERAL HOME:	POA/FAMILY MEMBER AND CONTACT INFO:	NAME:
PHONE NUMBER:		PHONE NUMBER:

CHECK ALL THAT APPLY :(SEE SUMMARY FOR FURTHER DETAILS)

☐ GLASSES   ☐ COAGS   ☐ DENTURES

☐ HEARING DISABILITY   ☐ DIABETES   ☐ THYROID

PATIENT NAME :		BIRTHDAY:		SOC :		HT :
DOCTOR NAME :		PHONE NUMBER:				
PMH PRIMARY DIAGNOSIS :						
MONTH						
KPS						
PPS						
WEIGHT						
BMI						
AMBUL- ATION						
BATHING						
TRANSFER						
RESPIRATORY						
CARDIAC						
SKIN						

FEEDING (INTAKE)					
SLEEP					
CONTINENCE					
COGNITION					
FALLS					
FAST SCORE					
INFECTIONS					
LABS APPOINTMENTS					

DAY:...../...../.....　　　　　　　　HOME HEALTH AID (HHA):

FUNERAL HOME:

PHONE NUMBER:

POA/FAMILY MEMBER AND CONTACT INFO:

NAME:

PHONE NUMBER:

CHECK ALL THAT APPLY :(SEE SUMMARY FOR FURTHER DETAILS)

☐ GLASSES　　　　☐ COAGS　　　　☐ DENTURES

☐ HEARING DISABILITY　　　　☐ DIABETES　　　　☐ THYROID

| PATIENT NAME : | | BIRTHDAY: | | SOC : | | HT : |
| DOCTOR NAME : | | PHONE NUMBER: | | | | |

PMH PRIMARY DIAGNOSIS :

MONTH						
KPS						
PPS						
WEIGHT						
BMI						
AMBUL-ATION						
BATHING						
TRANSFER						
RESPIRATORY						
CARDIAC						
SKIN						

FEEDING (INTAKE)					
SLEEP					
CONTINENCE					
COGNITION					
FALLS					
FAST SCORE					
INFECTIONS					
LABS APPOINTMENTS					

DAY:....../....../..... HOME HEALTH AID (HHA):

FUNERAL HOME:

PHONE NUMBER:

POA/FAMILY MEMBER AND CONTACT INFO:

NAME:

PHONE NUMBER:

CHECK ALL THAT APPLY : (SEE SUMMARY FOR FURTHER DETAILS)

☐ GLASSES ☐ COAGS ☐ DENTURES

☐ HEARING DISABILITY ☐ DIABETES ☐ THYROID

| PATIENT NAME : | | BIRTHDAY: | | SOC : | | HT : |
| DOCTOR NAME : | | PHONE NUMBER: | | | | |

PMH PRIMARY DIAGNOSIS :

MONTH						
KPS						
PPS						
WEIGHT						
BMI						
AMBUL-ATION						
BATHING						
TRANSFER						
RESPIRATORY						
CARDIAC						
SKIN						

FEEDING (INTAKE)					
SLEEP					
CONTINENCE					
COGNITION					
FALLS					
FAST SCORE					
INFECTIONS					
LABS APPOINTMENTS					

DAY:...../...../.....   HOME HEALTH AID (HHA):

FUNERAL HOME:

PHONE NUMBER:

POA/FAMILY MEMBER AND CONTACT INFO:

NAME:

PHONE NUMBER:

CHECK ALL THAT APPLY :(SEE SUMMARY FOR FURTHER DETAILS)

☐ GLASSES   ☐ COAGS   ☐ DENTURES

☐ HEARING DISABILITY   ☐ DIABETES   ☐ THYROID

PATIENT NAME :		BIRTHDAY:		SOC :		HT :
DOCTOR NAME :		PHONE NUMBER:				

PMH PRIMARY DIAGNOSIS :

MONTH						
KPS						
PPS						
WEIGHT						
BMI						
AMBUL-ATION						
BATHING						
TRANSFER						
RESPIRATORY						
CARDIAC						
SKIN						

FEEDING (INTAKE)					
SLEEP					
CONTINENCE					
COGNITION					
FALLS					
FAST SCORE					
INFECTIONS					
LABS APPOINTMENTS					

DAY:...../...../.....   HOME HEALTH AID (HHA):

FUNERAL HOME:

PHONE NUMBER:

POA/FAMILY MEMBER AND CONTACT INFO:

NAME:

PHONE NUMBER:

CHECK ALL THAT APPLY :(SEE SUMMARY FOR FURTHER DETAILS)

☐ GLASSES ☐ COAGS ☐ DENTURES

☐ HEARING DISABILITY ☐ DIABETES ☐ THYROID

| PATIENT NAME : | | BIRTHDAY: | | SOC : | | HT : |

DOCTOR NAME :   **PHONE NUMBER:**

PMH PRIMARY DIAGNOSIS :

MONTH						
KPS						
PPS						
WEIGHT						
BMI						
AMBUL-ATION						
BATHING						
TRANSFER						
RESPIRATORY						
CARDIAC						
SKIN						

FEEDING (INTAKE)						
SLEEP						
CONTINENCE						
COGNITION						
FALLS						
FAST SCORE						
INFECTIONS						
LABS APPOINTMENTS						

DAY:...../...../.....   HOME HEALTH AID (HHA):

FUNERAL HOME:

PHONE NUMBER:

POA/FAMILY MEMBER AND CONTACT INFO:

NAME:

PHONE NUMBER:

CHECK ALL THAT APPLY :(SEE SUMMARY FOR FURTHER DETAILS)

☐ GLASSES   ☐ COAGS   ☐ DENTURES

☐ HEARING DISABILITY ☐ DIABETES   ☐ THYROID

PATIENT NAME : BIRTHDAY: SOC : HT :

DOCTOR NAME : PHONE NUMBER:

PMH PRIMARY DIAGNOSIS :

MONTH						
KPS						
PPS						
WEIGHT						
BMI						
AMBUL-ATION						
BATHING						
TRANSFER						
RESPIRATORY						
CARDIAC						
SKIN						

FEEDING (INTAKE)						
SLEEP						
CONTINENCE						
COGNITION						
FALLS						
FAST SCORE						
INFECTIONS						
LABS APPOINTMENTS						

DAY:...../...../.....   HOME HEALTH AID (HHA):

FUNERAL HOME:

PHONE NUMBER:

POA/FAMILY MEMBER AND CONTACT INFO:

NAME:

PHONE NUMBER:

CHECK ALL THAT APPLY :(SEE SUMMARY FOR FURTHER DETAILS)

☐ GLASSES ☐ COAGS ☐ DENTURES

☐ HEARING DISABILITY ☐ DIABETES ☐ THYROID

| PATIENT NAME : | | BIRTHDAY: | | SOC : | | HT : |
| DOCTOR NAME : | | PHONE NUMBER: | | | | |

PMH PRIMARY DIAGNOSIS :

MONTH					
KPS					
PPS					
WEIGHT					
BMI					
AMBUL-ATION					
BATHING					
TRANSFER					
RESPIRATORY					
CARDIAC					
SKIN					

FEEDING (INTAKE)						
SLEEP						
CONTINENCE						
COGNITION						
FALLS						
FAST SCORE						
INFECTIONS						
LABS APPOINTMENTS						

DAY:...../...../.....   HOME HEALTH AID (HHA):

FUNERAL HOME:

PHONE NUMBER:

POA/FAMILY MEMBER AND CONTACT INFO:

NAME:

PHONE NUMBER:

CHECK ALL THAT APPLY :(SEE SUMMARY FOR FURTHER DETAILS)

☐ GLASSES   ☐ COAGS   ☐ DENTURES

☐ HEARING DISABILITY   ☐ DIABETES   ☐ THYROID

PATIENT NAME :		BIRTHDAY:		SOC :		HT :
DOCTOR NAME :		PHONE NUMBER:				

PMH PRIMARY DIAGNOSIS :

MONTH						
KPS						
PPS						
WEIGHT						
BMI						
AMBUL-ATION						
BATHING						
TRANSFER						
RESPIRATORY						
CARDIAC						
SKIN						

FEEDING (INTAKE)					
SLEEP					
CONTINENCE					
COGNITION					
FALLS					
FAST SCORE					
INFECTIONS					
LABS APPOINTMENTS					

DAY:...../...../.....   HOME HEALTH AID (HHA):

FUNERAL HOME:

PHONE NUMBER:

POA/FAMILY MEMBER AND CONTACT INFO:

NAME:

PHONE NUMBER:

CHECK ALL THAT APPLY :(SEE SUMMARY FOR FURTHER DETAILS)

☐ GLASSES   ☐ COAGS   ☐ DENTURES

☐ HEARING DISABILITY   ☐ DIABETES   ☐ THYROID